# Being anxious helps to achieve.

**leadership is a superpower**

**By**

# MIX LEONARD

# Table of content

**Introduction** This book shows How you can lead with confidence and power when you're feeling uneasy. When your thoughts and heart are racing, how can you inspire and motivate others? Where does the fear go if you try to be a strong leader by hiding Of sure, anxiety serves a purpose. It safeguards us against damage. Tigers and mastodons are no longer our main predators; instead, we must contend with threats to our self-worth, rejection by our friends, or defeat in a contest for superiority. Although the emotion of anxiety has evolved, its shape has not. In other words, even if predators no longer pursue people, we nevertheless experience the same neurological and bodily reactions when we worry about the health of our loved ones, whether we'll have a job next week or next year, or whether our firm will fail. Stress is a reaction to a situation's threat. Anxiety response to stress. Fear of the future is the root of anxiety. Sometimes that dread is justified, other times it is not. And occasionally, it concerns a future event. We were built for this moment, which is fantastic news for those of us who have long controlled our anxieties. Threats are interpreted differently by anxious persons, who use the brain's action-related regions. Whenever there is a threat, we act immediately. We might also feel more at ease in difficult situations. Anxiety, when used properly, can inspire us to increase the resourcefulness, productivity, and creativity of our teams. It can dismantle barriers and forge fresh connections.

Learning to recognize your anxiety in its various forms and manifestations is the first step. The second level involves taking action to control it daily and at trying times. Making wise choices and guiding people during stressful situations are required in the third level. The fourth stage entails creating a support system to assist you with long-term anxiety management. Recognizing and Embracing YourEmotions

So, worrying isn't pointless. The fear that keeps us awake at night during a financial crisis is usually able to help us come up with a plan to keep our companies operating. But if left unchecked, anxiety causes us to become distracted, drains our energy, and influences our decision-making. Since anxiety is a potent foe, we must make it our ally. You may still be a successful leader, regardless of whether you have an anxiety illness that has been diagnosed or this is your first experience with this powerful feeling. However, I'll be honest: If you don't confront your worry at some point, it will bring you down. Although difficult, doing this will improve both your life and your capacity to lead others.start today, in this very stressful.Learning to recognize your anxiety in its various forms and manifestations is the first step.

# Chapter1

## Over anxious ambition

Whatever stage of life we are in right now, we need to be aware of this truth. We traveled along a path to get here. Even though we may not have set out to arrive here, every one of us took a road to get to where we are now in life.

If you are experiencing fear and worry, you must have taken a path to get there. It might not have been done on purpose. Rarely is it. You followed a road that brought you here, and you must take a different path to leave behind fear and anxiety.

If your path has brought you to live in fear, worry, and anxiety... I'm happy to inform you! The direction you are going can be altered.

Fear is a sign that you are heading in the wrong direction. But you're not required to follow that course.

You have two options right now to alter your course and move in a different direction. These two things won't set you back any money either.

## MOST CHANGE DOESN'T TAKE PLACE RIGHT AWAY.

We must leave on foot. The difference, however, is that we can alter the course we are currently on.

I was a young child with excessive ambition. I wanted to finish all of my tests before anyone else and obtain the best grade in the class. I was so focused on doing well that my parents didn't even need to set a curfew for me because they could usually find me studying rather than going out on a Friday night. Everything seemed to be going well for me, at least until I started college and had my first encounter with my anxiety problem.

I had all these goals in mind for my life, but because my anxiety was interfering with daily living, I wasn't able to accomplish them as I had hoped. I would cry from stress every time I sat down to study for an exam or got ready for an interview for an internship. Either I'd have a full-blown anxiety attack and be unable to leave the house, or I'd arrive drenched in sweat, my eyes swollen shut, and my fingers bloody and gouged. The treatment I eventually received has helped over the years, but it can sometimes be challenging to get things done when anxiety hangs over your head.

This conflict between worry and aspiration is rather typical for those with mental illnesses.No matter how paralyzing anxiety may feel at any particular time, it doesn't have to break your resolve. Anxiety causes people to doubt their abilities and makes them scared to try to attain their goals because the fear of failure is so overwhelming. How to be ambitious when you're feeling anxious.

Don't Ignore Your Worry

Anxiety disorder sufferers frequently "fear the increased responsibilities and expectations of success." You could get a sense of being stuck and out of control whenever you approach or even consider attaining something.

Remember that fighting off your nervous feelings only serves to exacerbate your condition. Do not brush off your worry as unnecessary or stupid.

Recognize your apprehensions and permit yourself a brief period of anxiety. The first step to making progress is simply naming your anxiety, whether it be verbally expressed or experienced inside.

Without any type of organization or punctuation, jot down every nervous thought you have about the future. Even if you never go back and read it, simply getting it down in writing will feel good. How to Handle Your Ambition When It Makes You Anxious There is always a hint of nervousness there in chats with people regarding their professions. A lot of people talk about the moment when "everything will fall into place" because they have reached a goal. It could be a graduation, getting a certain job, getting promoted, launching a nonprofit, or making a whole career change. However, I've observed that they frequently become immobile and fail to recognize the changes that are already present because they are concerned about their advancement. As they wait for the significant milestone, they are simply going about their everyday business. Despite being exceedingly analytical and worried, I learned how to control my anxieties and preoccupations during transitional periods. You must adhere to these principles and practices if you want to control your anxiety while pursuing your profession and your ambitions.

## What's Motivating You: Ambition vs. Anxiety?

**Anxiety can pass for a variety of important-sounding traits, including**

thoughtful people-pleaser, meticulous planner, and one of my personal favorites, ambitious go-getter.

I can't even begin to count how many people I've met who tightly conceal their anxieties under a façade of ambition. They frequently spend too much time working, drinking, or eating, and barely get any sleep.

I have visited there. In large part because I thought anxiety was my only genuine power and talent, and that underneath that, I wasn't worth much at all, I used to think that my anxiety was the only thing that made my ambition function, the only thing that was going to take me forward.

If you hadn't been concerned about what people thought of you, where would you be now? If you had done it slightly differently or listened, you might have succeeded. Without someone bugging you about it and blaming you for your mistakes, you would never have completed that task.

You must understand the differences between worry and ambition if you want to recover your self-worth and acknowledge your abilities and value.

angst is...

Every pore is filled with anxiety as fret about details that nobody else seems to be aware of.

a persistent need for tranquility amidst worry.

Desire is...

the desire to accomplish significant goals, the motivation to turn your aspirations into reality, and the unwavering dedication to take wonderful care of oneself while making every effort to meet one's goals.

Fear says...

"Get moving, sleep is for losers; if you don't push yourself to the absolute limit to achieve perfection, you're going to fail."

"They all know you're faking it; show them you know what you're doing, put on that smile, and start selling," the person said.

"Why should anyone ever trust you? Never know what to say, do, or who to be.

Desire says...

Failure is a necessary ingredient in the success recipe; if you keep trying new things, you'll discover what the other components are.

Be yourself; nobody is an expert at everything; successful individuals are those that try their best nonetheless and pick things up along the way. You can do this.

First and foremost, have faith in your abilities and determination to succeed.

How does anxiousness feel?

heart-pounding, a tornado of racing thoughts, sweaty hands, a tingling sense of dread, and the feeling that your gut is being crushed by a thousand pounds.

**Desire feels like...**

butterflies doing the dance, which is both enjoyable and unsettling, and a revitalizing energy that pushes you through sensations of overwhelm.

To choose the least objectionable course of action, anxiety compels you to consider every eventuality that could result from a single action, including what other people will think and feel.

But don't ponder this too much! You need to act immediately since time is important; otherwise, the end of the world will likely come quickly.

Consider the action you made, how it probably affected everyone nearby, how they feel about you and the action, and how likely it is that, on a scale of 1 to 10, everyone now despises you.

utterly exhausted and take a nap.

Desire drives you...

Make a plan to accomplish that goal by breaking it down into smaller goals after weighing your options and selecting the one that makes the most sense to you right now.

Invest in the tools that will enable you to accomplish that objective (real tools, not just three brand-new, posh notebooks from Target that you will only ever use for the first five pages before putting them in a box and wondering why you can't make bullet journaling work for you; or maybe that's just me).

**Celebrate your accomplishments and consider your future goals.
Ambition versus worry.**

Avoiding anxious circumstances can make them worse! According to experts, it's a typical response to stressful circumstances, but if a person doesn't work to overcome it, it will only get worse. There are various alternatives to utilizing prescription medications for the treatment of anxiety.

By making changes to their nutrition, increasing their quality of sleep, and engaging in daily exercise, a person can reduce certain symptoms of anxiety.

Reducing the body's consumption of sugar and processed meals helps lower inflammation, which in turn lowers anxiety levels.

It is also known that getting between seven and nine hours of sleep each night and doing about two and a half hours of moderate exercise each week will help reduce symptoms. For daily pressures, such as needing to meet a deadline at work or feeling under pressure for another cause, mindfulness, and meditation can be used to manage them.

breathing awareness, in which a person concentrates on their breath, slows it down, and as a result calms themselves.

Avoidance is a bad method to deal with worry and could make things worse as a result.

While avoiding situations that you know would make you stressed out can be effective in some circumstances, you can't protect yourself from these problems indefinitely. Avoidance has a bit of a two-pronged effect. An individual with social anxiety may occasionally experience anxiety attacks brought on by being around people or having to perform."The longer you put off doing those things, the greater the anxiety grows, and the tougher it is to carry out some of these necessary actions."If you work, you can't always stay silent in meetings."

If you were to witness me going about my days and take a peek at my life, you probably wouldn't notice that I'm anxious unless you know what to look for. a driven, focused, organized, aspirational, high achiever, and one who keeps everything under control under duress. proactive, helpful, dependable, and outstanding. Being a high achiever indicates that you excelled in all facets of your life and received First Class Honors. Being an ambitious person, I poured myself into starting my own business. You become a great coach if you can read people. Being the proactive one entails always being the festival-going friend who is prepared, the one who makes dinner reservations, and the one who decides how to divide the tab. Being driven entails advancing your education at all times, engaging in professional growth, and striving to be "the best you can be." You are the best if you are the most organized. You are highly self-sufficient and always know where you are headed. Of course, these actions will influence a person's life; success may be greatly attributed to this way of being. But pay attention—it will also cost you a lot Because there is a persistent discomfort beneath the surface. Constantly feeling the desire to exert control over your environment for your well-being. You can deal with anything if you are ready. You can unwind if others are taken care of. If you succeed, you will receive affection and adulation in return. I have complete power over all you have.

Only so much pressure can we withstand. We eventually tilt over the brink when it becomes too much. How can we go when so many of our anxious features help us but also have the potential to be our undoing?

Over the past five years, I've put a lot of time, money, and effort into learning to achieve the balance between these two. I've tried counseling, talk therapy, medication, mindfulness training, herbal medicines, diet modifications, and coaching.

I've given myself some time to think about how my upbringing influenced the characteristics I observe in myself today. It's crucial to realize that, on some level, we develop behaviors that work for us. Our sole purpose as children is to learn how to survive, therefore any actions that resulted in our receiving more affection, consideration, care, food, drink, or shelter were likely reinforced. Let me be clear: I was raised by two devoted, thoughtful, and watchful parents. I never felt lacking in anything. I was never mistreated or neglected.

But thanks to all the elders in my life, I've learned the value of success, preparation, and character. what made me more lovable and popular. I discovered the benefits of happiness and the virtue of looking out for other people. Over time, I continued to practice these habits. These habits are still rewarded because they still garner social acceptance today. You will become more self-aware in situations where you might have previously reflexively engaged in these actions if you understand the relationship between environment and behavior.

## Developing coping mechanisms to lessen the physiological impacts of anxiety

I get in my head when I'm anxious. When I become aware of this, I understand that I need to accept my feelings and permit myself to be in them. According to research, attempting to avoid, decrease, or combat anxiety (including emotions and ideas) just makes the experience worse. We keep having the same experience, which can be more upsetting. Simply saying out loud, "I'm noticing the feeling of anxiety," is my first step. I'm conscious of the concept that.

While doing this, I'm gently bringing myself back to the present moment and into my body rather than remaining in my head (it can be challenging to achieve a balance between presence and not avoiding one's thoughts). By taking several long, calm, deep breaths into my abdomen, I'm turning off my sympathetic nervous system (fight/flight/freeze) and turning on my parasympathetic nervous system.

**Increasing behavioral adaptability and selecting substitute behaviors as necessary.**

After practicing mindful breathing, it becomes simpler to decide on a habit that will benefit you over the long term. It can be simpler to select fresh responses when you are conscious of what you're doing and the results you're after. I have the option to choose flawed action over perfectionism, tiny steps over inaction, and self-care over working through fatigue. These habits, which are in line with my objectives and beliefs, can be reinforced in a variety of ways. Some of these actions may reinforce themselves just by how good they make me feel when I do them. Keep telling yourself that you are secure, loved, and worthwhile throughout everything.

You can still be ambitious by making these decisions. you who are determined. the high-achieving you, BUT you may be her without teetering dangerously close to the edge of anxiety-inducing

overthinking, overdoing, and overcompensation.
You will regain your equilibrium through these decisions as you delicately dance between ambition and anxiety.

Worrying implies responsibility.

Those who worry constantly think that worrying is equivalent to being "responsible."
believes that you would not consider yourself to be a responsible person if you did not spend so much time worrying about anything.
As a result, you will visit the doctor every month to make sure that you

have not caught the most recent flu strain.

You have to believe that is what any responsible person would demand, so you insist on these periodic examinations. must suffice, just in case.

## Chapter 2

## DON'T STRESS OVER IT.

I call those who worry excessively "what-if thinkers," or people who act in "just-in-case scenarios."
Not only do worry-prone people hold certain views about the harmful effects that worry causes, but they also support the ideas that worry has positive effects.

The issue is that these good ideas about the worrying process overwhelm their negative beliefs about how worrying works.

Those who worry a lot compare worrying too:
· Raising one's defenses
• Being more ready for foreseeable traumatic life occurrences
• Lessening one's sense of threat when confronted with the unexpected.
"Don't worry about it," when said to a warrior, is seen as a sign that they should lower their guard.
What occurs when someone lowers their guard? They become worried and aroused, which causes them to feel vulnerable and overestimate the

threat. As a result, they exhibit reassurance-seeking behaviors to calm themselves down.

## CONFRONT YOUR ANXIETY BELIEFS

Instead of telling someone to "don't worry about it," I advise you to help them (or yourself) change how anxious thoughts are perceived.

The next time you have this thought, remember to challenge the idea that worrying will stop bad things from happening by asking yourself: "Have there been times in the past when I've effectively dealt with an unexpected crisis without worrying about it before it occurred?"

What if you questioned yourself, "Do I have friends who I consider to be responsible individuals, and do I view them as people who worry as much as I do?" to the notion that worrying equals being a responsible person? Other ideas that contribute to the persistence of chronic worry include:

• Solving problems is the same as worrying,

• If I worry, it will make it easier for me to deal with negative feelings like sadness or rage should they truly come true.

• My worry serves as a driving force for action.

The worry process is a love/hate relationship, a two-edged sword. Give up your hate and embrace your love.

## Chapter 3

**Unhealthy approach and bad behavior.**

Start today to eliminate them from your life. When you do, you'll open up room for new habits to take their place. It doesn't take much, Consistent effort is the key.
Start chasing the right things instead of running after what's wrong. problems are not something to be ashamed of or avoid, it's an opportunities to learn and grow.

Everyone makes mistakes, but it's up to you whether you'll give them the power to keep you from doing what you want. find your strength.

make them work for you. Control is an illusion. Don't try to control everything, you will quickly become frustrated and angry. remember the only thing you can reliably control is your reaction to the things going on around you and within you.

The way to be happy is to be accountable for your actions and responsible for your consequences.

What choices can you make to start creating happiness? Did you wake up in bed? Don't take the necessities of life for granted. Be grateful for all of life's blessings: food, health, relationships, your mind, and your heart. At the end of the day, quit the habits that do not serve you…

Whatever the bad habit is that you are looking to break, visualize yourself crushing it.

enjoying your success.

that will show you how to make the change.

When does your bad habit happen?

## Chapter 4

## Controlling the bad habit

## How to Stop an Addiction

There is nothing wrong with habits; Some are quite helpful, like when you automatically switch off the lights when you leave a room or set out your clothing the night before work.

It might take time to break bad habits, especially when you have been doing them for a while.

## establishing a habit

Several ideas exist about the formation of habits.

## Routine

This is the action that the trigger is linked to. While nervousness causes you to bite your nails, flushing the toilet causes you to wash your hands.

Routine behavior can develop through repeated actions.

## Reward

When you do something that makes you happy or makes you feel better, your brain releases dopamine, making you want to do it again.

It can be difficult to break bad habits, especially when you have been doing it for a long time. But a better grasp of how habits begin helps make the process easier.

establishing a habit

Several ideas exist about the formation of habits.

Reminder

**This is a trigger or cue, and it might be a conscious action like flushing the toilet, or it might be a sensation like anxiety.**

**Routine**

**This is the action that the trigger is linked to. While nervousness causes you to bite your nails, flushing the toilet causes you to wash your hands. Routine behavior can develop through repeated actions.**
**Reward.**
**A behavior's related reward also aids in the development of habits. When**

you do something that makes you happy or makes you feel better, your brain releases dopamine, making you want to do it again.

Track your habit for a few days to determine whether it exhibits any trends.

Note details such as:

When does the routine conduct occur?

When in the day?

How does it make you feel at the time?

Exist, other participants?

Does it follow another event immediately?

You can become more aware of your thoughts, feelings, and actions by practicing mindfulness. Simply monitoring impulses related to your habit without passing judgment on them or responding to them is this practice.

It might be simpler for you to consider different options when you become more conscious of these repetitive actions and the triggers that cause them, such as ignoring reminder cues or acting otherwise.

Change the behavior by adopting a new one.

trying to replace the undesirable activity

With a new behavior rather than just trying to cease the undesirable behavior, you could find it easier to break the habit.

Let's say you are used to eating candy and you want to stop eating it. If all you do is try, just stop and control your appetite. However, find another snack choice, that way stopping it will be easy.

# Chapter 5

anxiety that comes from social life.

social phobia.

A persistent and severe fear of social situations is referred to as social anxiety disorder.

It's a typical issue that typically manifests in adolescence. It may be upsetting and significantly affect your life.

Some people find that as they grow older, things get better. But for others, it continues after receiving no treatment.

It's advisable to seek assistance if you experience signs. You can manage it with the help of therapies.

Social anxiety symptoms

**Shyness is not the same as social anxiety. It's a persistent worry that interferes with day-to-day activities.**
**Most people worry about social settings on occasion, but those who have social anxiety worry excessively before, during, and after them.**

**If you avoid or worry a lot about social activities like group chats, eating with company, and parties, such as meeting strangers, striking up conversations, speaking on the phone,**

working, or shopping, you may have social anxiety.

Always be concerned about doing something you believe to be embarrassing, such as blushing, perspiring, or acting incompetent, and find it challenging to perform tasks while others are present. You can always feel like people are watching and judging you, fear criticism, avoid eye contact, or lack confidence.

frequently have symptoms including feeling queasy, perspiring, shaking, or a racing heartbeat; have panic attacks where you experience intense dread and worry that last only a short time;

Many persons who suffer from social anxiety also struggle with depression, generalized anxiety disorder, or panic disorder.

When to seek social anxiety treatment Checking for social anxiety is a smart practice, especially if it's significantly affecting your life.

It's a common issue, and there are solutions available.

Asking for assistance can be challenging, but those who provide it are aware that a lot of individuals experience social anxiety and will work to make you feel at ease.

To learn more about your social anxiety, they will probe you about your emotions, actions, and symptoms.

If they suspect social anxiety, they will refer you to a mental health professional so they may do a thorough evaluation and discuss available therapies. Which, if you truly want to be yourself and get rid of such anxiousness, you won't need it.

Strategies for overcoming social anxiety

Self-care can help with social anxiety and may be a good starting point before pursuing other treatments.

trick that work

Try some relaxation techniques, like breathing exercises for stress, to help you feel more at ease in challenging situations. Break up difficult situations into smaller parts and work on feeling more relaxed with each part. Focus on what people are saying rather than automatically assuming the worst. You are your solution, and it all starts with you.